Copycat Thai Recipes

Learn to Cook 50 Recipes from the
Most Famous Thai Restaurants

By

Sommario

3

Introduction

Welcome to this fantastic culinary journey to Eastern, Thai cuisine.

I will try to teach you as much as possible, with tips and fantastic recipes, easy and fast within the reach of even the most novice cooks.

In this book, you will find a comprehensive approach to cook Thai dishes at home. The recipes are quite simple, and with minimal effort from your side, you can taste the actual essence of Thai cuisine.

There are plenty of books on this subject on the market, thanks again for choosing this one! Every effort was made to ensure it is full of as much useful information as possible, and please enjoy it!

Chapter 1: Rice And Noodles Recipes

One-Pot Rice Noodles

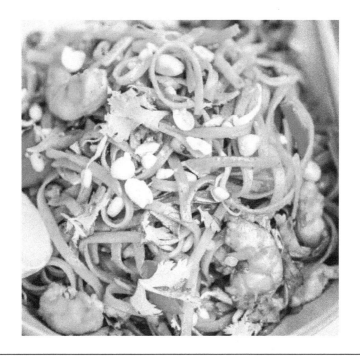

Total Prep & Cooking Time: Forty minutes

Yields: Four servings

Nutrition Facts: Calories: 576.2 | Protein: 15.4g | Carbs: 96.4g | Fat: 9.1g | Fiber: 3.7g

Ingredients

- Two tbsps. of cornstarch
- One and a half tbsp. of water
- Six cups of chicken stock
- Three tbsps. of soy sauce
- One tbsp. of fish sauce
- Half tbsp. of rice vinegar
- One-third tbsp. of chili-garlic sauce
- Two tsps. of each
- Garlic (minced)
- Vegetable oil
- Ginger (minced)
- One tsp. of coriander (ground)
- Sixteen ounces of rice noodles
- One cup of each
- Red bell pepper (sliced)
- Zucchini (sliced)
- Two breasts of chicken (cooked, cut in small cubes)

- Half cup of each

- Cilantro (chopped)

- Peanuts (crushed)

Method:

1.   Combine the cornstarch along with some water in a cup. Combine the mixture of cornstarch with chicken stock, fish sauce, soy sauce, chili-garlic sauce, rice vinegar, garlic, ginger, vegetable oil, and coriander. Boil the mixture.

2.   Add the rice noodles in the sauce and simmer for ten minutes until the noodles are tender. Add red bell pepper, zucchini, and cubes of chicken. Boil the mixture and simmer for five minutes.

3.   Serve with cilantro and peanuts from the top.

Thai Pesto Noodles

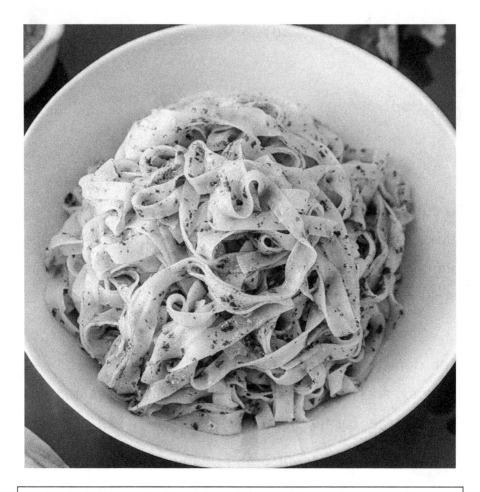

Total Prep & Cooking Time: Twenty minutes

Yields: Four servings

Nutrition Facts: Calories: 112 | Protein: 5.9g | Carbs: 8.9g | Fat: 9.8g | Fiber: 1.6g

Ingredients

- Ten ounces of rice noodles (thick)
- One bunch of cilantro
- One-fourth cup of peanut butter
- Three garlic cloves (minced)
- Three tbsps. of olive oil (extra virgin)
- Two tbsps. of ginger (minced)
- One and a half tbsp. of fish sauce
- One tbsp. of brown sugar
- Half tsp. of cayenne pepper

Method:

1. Soak the rice noodles in warm water. Soak them for about ten minutes. Let the noodles sit until tender.

2. In the meantime, combine peanut butter, olive oil, garlic, ginger, brown sugar, fish sauce, and pepper in a food processor. Keep blending until smooth.

3. Heat some oil in a wok. Add the pesto sauce. Cook for one minute. Add the soaked noodles and toss them for combining. Cook for one minute.

4. Serve hot.

Thai Noodle Curry Bowl

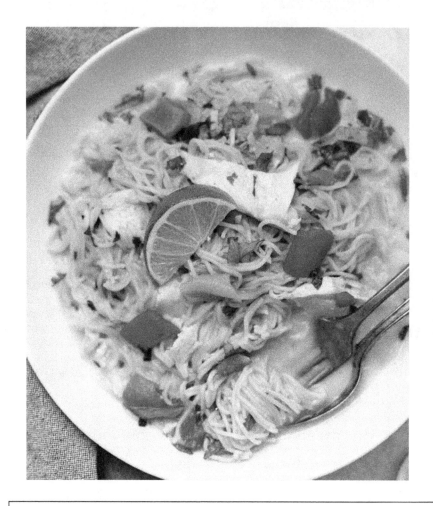

Total Prep & Cooking Time: Thirty minutes

Yields: Six servings

Nutrition Facts: Calories: 208.3 | Protein: 3.4g | Carbs: 37.2g | Fat: 4.7g | Fiber: 1.7g

Ingredients

- One tbsp. of peanut oil

- Two garlic cloves (minced)

- Thirty ounces of Thai ginger broth

- One carrot (cut in matchsticks)

- Eight ounces of rice noodles (thick, cooked)

- Three tbsps. of green onions (sliced)

- One-third cup of cilantro (chopped)

- Two tbsps. of peanuts (chopped)

- Six lime wedges

Method:

1.   Heat some oil in a pot. Add the garlic. Stir-fry for thirty seconds.

2.   Add the ginger broth and boil. Add the sliced carrots and cook them for five minutes.

3.   Add the cooked noodles and simmer for four minutes.

4.   Serve the curry noodles in serving bowls with cilantro, peanuts, and green onions from the top.

Pas See Ew (Noodles With Broccoli and Beef)

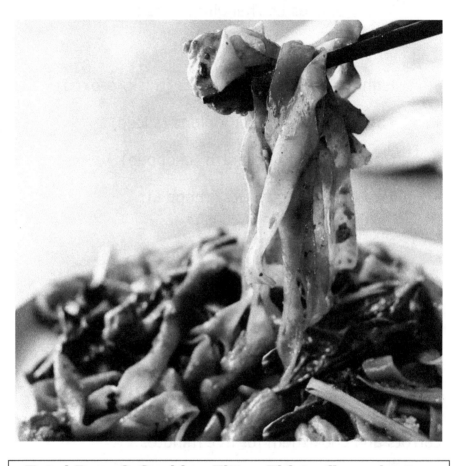

Total Prep & Cooking Time: Thirty-five minutes

Yields: Eight servings

Nutrition Facts: Calories: 182.3 | Protein: 5.7g |
Carbs: 24.7g | Fat: 5.9g | Fiber: 0.9g

Ingredients

- Eight ounces of thick rice noodles
- One cup of broccoli (cut in bite-size pieces)
- One tbsp. of vegetable oil
- One tsp. of garlic (crushed)
- Half pound of rib-eye steak (thinly sliced)
- Half cup of water
- One and a half tbsp. of cornstarch
- Three tbsps. of each
- Soy sauce
- Oyster sauce
- Two tbsps. of each
- White sugar
- Fish sauce
- Half tsp. of each
- Black pepper (ground)
- Salt
- One large egg

Method:

1.   Place the noodles in a large bowl. Cover it using hot water. Soak the noodles for ten minutes. Drain the water and keep aside.

2.   Boil water in a small pot. Add the pieces of broccoli and cook for seven minutes until firm. Drain the water and keep aside.

3.   Heat the oil in a large skillet. Add the garlic. Cook for three minutes and add the steak. Cook for seven minutes until the meat pieces are tender.

4.   Combine the cornstarch along with some water in a bowl. Add the mixture to the skillet. Add soy sauce, oyster sauce, sugar, and fish sauce. Stir the mixture.

5.   Add the broccoli along with the noodles. Add pepper and salt for seasoning.

6.   Cook the egg in another skillet.

7.   Add the cooked eggs to the noodles and mix well.

8.   Serve hot.

Spicy Peanut Noodles

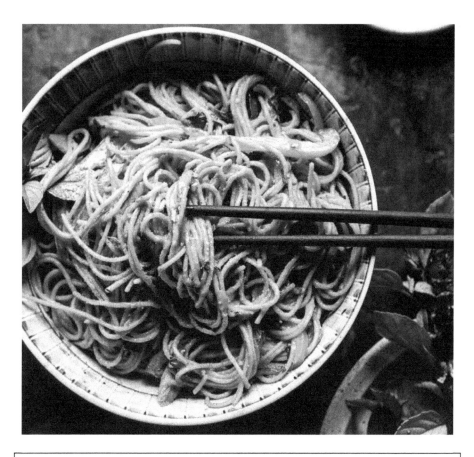

Total Prep & Cooking Time: Thirty-five minutes

Yields: Six servings

Nutrition Facts: Calories: 680.2 | Protein: 25.7g |
Carbs: 80.3g | Fat: 27.2g | Fiber: 5.7g

Ingredients

For the sauce:

- Half cup of peanut butter

- Six tbsps. of soy sauce

- Three tbsps. of each

- Rice vinegar

- Brown sugar

- Sesame oil

- Two red chilies (chopped)

- Two tbsps. of each

- Ginger (grated)

- Chili-garlic sauce

- One tsp. of fish sauce

- Half tsp. of black pepper (ground)

For the noodles:

- Three tbsps. of olive oil

- One pound of chicken breast (cut in cubes of three-fourth inch)

- One cup of carrots (cut in matchsticks)

- One red bell pepper (sliced in strips)

- Four green onions (sliced)

- Two cups of bean sprouts (rinsed)

- One-fourth cup of cilantro (chopped)

- Sixteen ounces of rice noodles

- One tbsp. of peanuts (chopped)

Method:

1. Whisk all the listed ingredients for the sauce in a bowl. Keep aside.

2. Take a large wok and heat two tbsps. of oil in it. Add the pieces of chicken and cook for three minutes. Add one-fourth cup of the sauce to the chicken. Cook for two minutes. Transfer the cooked chicken along with the juices in a bowl.

3. Heat the leftover oil and add the carrots. Cook for three minutes and add the bell peppers. Cook for one minute. Add the chicken, green onions, remaining sauce, cilantro, and bean sprouts. Cook the mixture for one minute.

4.   Cover the noodles with hot water for five minutes. Drain the water and add the cooked noodles to the mixture.

5.   Add the peanuts and stir-fry for two minutes.

6.   Serve the noodles with peanuts from the top.

Pad Kee Mao (Thai Drunken Noodles)

Total Prep & Cooking Time: Thirty-five minutes

Yields: Four servings

Nutrition Facts: Calories: 567.3 | Protein: 7.3g | Carbs: 106.3g | Fat: 12.2g | Fiber: 4.6g

Ingredients

- One pound of rice noodles (dried)

- Three tbsps. of oil

- One-fourth cup of each

- Thai chilies

- Onion (sliced)

- Two tbsps. of each

- Garlic (minced)

- Soy sauce

- Fish sauce

- One tbsp. of brown sugar

- One red bell pepper (cut in pieces of one inch)

- One cup of each

- Peapods

- Broccoli (chopped)

- Half cup of carrots (chopped)

- One-third cup of basil (chopped)

Method:

1.   Add the noodles in a pot and cover with hot water. Add one tbsp. of oil to the noodles and soak for ten minutes. Drain the water and keep aside.

2.   Take a large wok and heat the oil in it. Add the onion, chilies, and garlic. Fry the mixture for five minutes. Add the fish sauce, brown sugar, and soy sauce. Stir the mixture. Add the noodles, broccoli, bell pepper, carrots, and pea pods. Stir-fry the mixture for five minutes. Add the basil.

3.   Serve the noodles with basil from the top.

Thai Noodle Pork Bowl

Total Prep & Cooking Time: Thirty minutes

Yields: Six servings

Nutrition Facts: Calories: 590.3 | Protein: 21.5g | Carbs: 44.6g | Fat: 36.5g | Fiber: 4.9g

Ingredients

- Twelve ounces of rice noodles (wide)

- One-fourth cup of soy sauce

- One tbsp. of each

- Vegetable oil

- Honey

- Ginger paste

- Garlic (chopped)

- Two tsps. of fish sauce

- Two tbsps. of red curry paste

- One can of coconut milk

- Two pounds of pork loin chops (cut in thin strips)

- One cup of carrots (julienned)

- Eight ounces of sugar snap peas

- One-third cup of cilantro (chopped)

- Half lime (juiced and zested)

Method:

1. Boil water in a large pot. Add some oil. Add the noodles and cook for two minutes. Drain the water and keep aside.

2. Whisk honey, soy sauce, and fish sauce in a bowl.

3. Take an iron skillet and add some oil in it. Add the ginger paste, garlic, and curry paste. Cook for one minute. Add the coconut milk and cook for one minute.

4. Add the strips of pork, peas, and carrots. Cook for five minutes. Add the mixture of soy sauce. Simmer the mixture for five minutes. Add the noodles and stir for one minute.

5. Serve the noodles hot with lime zest, lime juice, and cilantro from the top.

Rad Na Noodles

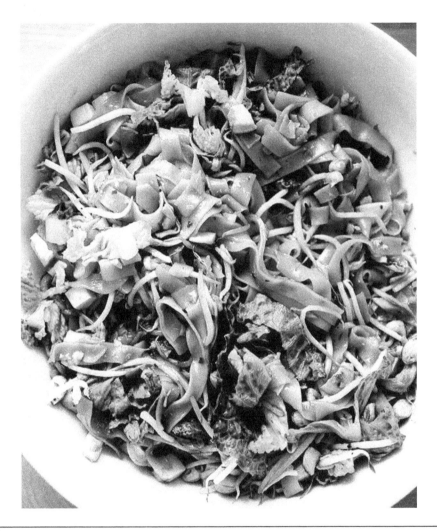

Total Prep & Cooking Time: Thirty minutes

Yields: Four servings

Nutrition Facts: Calories: 310.3 | Protein: 12.6g | Carbs: 35.9g | Fat: 13.6g | Fiber: 2.9g

Ingredients

- Two large eggs (beaten)

- Three tbsps. of each

- Fish sauce

- Soy sauce

- Brown sugar

- Rice vinegar

- One head of romaine lettuce

- Half tsp. of pepper flakes

- Six scallions (sliced)

- Half pound of bean sprouts

- One cup of peanuts (chopped)

- Eight ounces of rice noodles (wide)

- Two tbsps. of vegetable oil

- Hot sauce (for serving)

Method:

1.   Start by cooking the noodles in hot water for five minutes. Drain the water and keep aside.

2.   Whisk together fish sauce, soy sauce, rice vinegar, brown sugar, and three tbsps. of water in a bowl.

3.   Slice the lettuce into pieces of half an inch. Heat some oil in a large wok. Add the pepper flakes. Add the noodles and coat in oil. Add the prepared sauce toss for one minute.

4.   Cook the eggs as omelet in a skillet. Slice the omelet into thin slices.

5.   Add the eggs, scallions, nuts, and bean sprouts to the noodles. Cook for one minute.

6.   Serve hot with hot sauce from the top.

Creamy Thai Noodles

Total Prep & Cooking Time: Forty-five minutes

Yields: Four servings

Nutrition Facts: Calories: 336.3 | Protein: 12g | Carbs: 49.6g | Fat: 10.7g | Fiber: 4.9g

Ingredients

- Eight ounces of noodles

- One tbsp. of vegetable oil

- One tsp. of ginger (grated)

- Two garlic cloves (minced)

- Half cup of carrot (julienned)

- Two cups of cabbage (sliced)

- One-fourth cup of bean sprouts

- Cilantro, green onions, and peanuts (for garnishing)

For the sauce:

- Half cup of chicken stock
- Two tbsps. of each
- Soy sauce
- Peanut butter (creamy)
- One tsp. of sriracha
- Two tsps. of sesame oil
- One tbsp. of brown sugar
- One-fourth tsp. of red pepper flakes

Method:

1.	Combine the listed ingredients for the sauce in a bowl. Keep aside.

2.	Cook the noodles in boiling water for five minutes. Drain the water and keep aside.

3.	Add oil in a wok and cook the garlic along with the ginger.

4.   Add cabbage and carrots. Cook for three minutes. Add the prepared sauce and simmer for three minutes.

5.   Add the noodles along with the bean sprouts. Toss well for two minutes.

6.   Serve the noodles with cilantro, peanuts, and green onions from the top.

Rainbow Veggie Pad Thai

Total Prep & Cooking Time: Twenty minutes

Yields: Four servings

Nutrition Facts: Calories: 323.3 | Protein: 7.8g | Carbs: 35.7g | Fat: 16.7g | Fiber: 3.7g

Ingredients

- Four ounces of brown rice noodles
- One zucchini
- One red bell pepper
- Two carrots
- Half an onion
- Two tbsps. of oil
- One large egg (beaten)
- Half cup of peanuts (chopped)
- One cup of fresh herbs (green onions, cilantro, and basil)

For the sauce:

- Three tbsps. of each

- Fish sauce

- Chicken stock

- Brown sugar

- Two tbsps. of white vinegar

- One tbsp. of soy sauce

- One tsp. of chili paste

Method:

1.   Start by spiralizing the veggies using a spiralizer or a peeler. In case you do not have a peeler, you can cut them into thin strips.

2.   Add the ingredients of the sauce in a bowl and combine.

3.   Take a wok and heat some oil in it. Add the vegetables and cook for two minutes. Transfer the veggies to a bowl.

4.   Cook the noodles in hot water for five minutes. Drain the water. Add the noodles to the wok.

5.   Add the prepared sauce and toss the noodles. Push the noodles to one side and break the egg in the center. Scramble the egg. Combine it with the noodles.

6.   Add the cooked vegetables to the wok and stir-fry for two minutes. Add the herbs.

7.   Serve hot.

Thai Garlic and Ginger Noodle Bowl

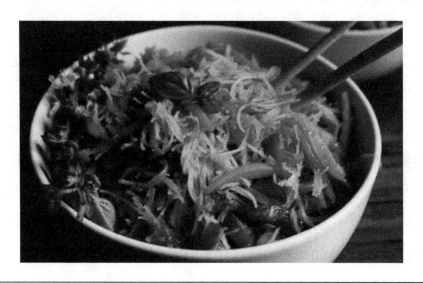

Total Prep & Cooking Time: Forty-five minutes

Yields: Four servings

Nutrition Facts: Calories: 389.3 | Protein: 7.8g | Carbs: 68.6g | Fat: 10.3g | Fiber: 9.3g

Ingredients

- Eight ounces of rice noodles

- Ten ounces of snow peas

- Two tbsps. of sesame oil

- Two tsps. of ginger (grated)

- One tbsp. of garlic (minced)

- Two cups of carrots (julienned)

- Five cups of cabbage (cut in bite-size pieces)

- Five ounces of shitake mushrooms (sliced in quarters, steamed)

For the sauce:

- Half cup of vegetable stock

- One tbsp. of sesame oil

- Two tbsps. of tamari

- Half tbsp. of coconut sugar

- One-third tsp. of each

- Sea salt

- Pepper flakes

Method:

1. Soak the noodles in hot water for about five minutes. Drain the water and keep aside.

2.   Blanch the snow peas in a pot of water for two minutes. Trim the ends before blanching. Drain the water and keep aside.

3.   Whisk the listed ingredients for the sauce in a small bowl. Keep aside.

4.   Take a large wok and heat some oil in it. Add the garlic and ginger. Cook for thirty seconds and add the mushrooms. Cook for one minute. Add the carrots and cabbage. Cook for two minutes. Keep the veggies aside along with the peas.

5.   Add the sauce in the wok and simmer for two minutes. Add the noodles and toss for coating.

6.   Add the vegetable mix and stir for two minutes.

7.   Serve the noodles hot.

Chapter 2: Meat and Poultry Recipes

Chicken and Pineapple Curry

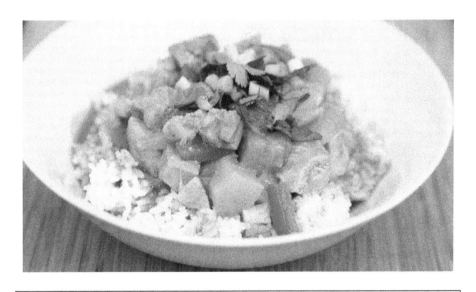

Total Prep & Cooking Time: Fifty minutes
Yields: Six servings
Nutrition Facts: Calories: 620.3 | Protein: 21.6g | Carbs: 74.7g | Fat: 35.4g | Fiber: 4.5g

Ingredients

- One-fourth cup of red curry paste

- Two cans of coconut milk

- Two breasts of chicken (cut in strips)

- Three tbsps. of fish sauce

- One-fourth cup of white sugar

- One and a half cup of bamboo shoots (sliced)

- Half a red bell pepper (julienned)

- Half a green bell pepper (julienned)

- One onion (chopped)

- One cup of pineapple chunks

Method:

1. Whisk together the curry paste along with one can of coconut milk. Add this mixture to the wok.

2. Add the remaining coconut milk along with fish sauce, chicken, bamboo shoots, and sugar. Boil for fifteen minutes.

3.   Add green bell pepper, onion, and red bell pepper in the wok. Cook for ten minutes.

4.   Add the pineapples and let the chicken sit for two minutes.

5.   Serve hot.

Thai Chicken Tenders

Total Prep & Cooking Time: Twelve minutes
Yields: Five servings
**Nutrition Facts: Calories: 349.3	Protein: 26.6g	Carbs: 15.9g	Fat: 20.1g	Fiber: 3.7g**

Ingredients

- Two tbsps. of sesame oil

- One pound of chicken (boneless, cut in strips)

- Two tsps. of ginger (minced)

- Half cup of hoisin sauce

- One cup of peanut butter (creamy)

- One tsp. of cayenne pepper

- One-third cup of scallions (chopped)

Method:

1.   Heat the oil in a large skillet. Add the chicken. Cook for three minutes.

2.   Add the hoisin sauce, ginger, peanut butter, and cayenne pepper. Cook for two minutes.

3.   Sprinkle scallions from the top and stir.

4.   Serve hot.

Thai-Style Barbeque Chicken

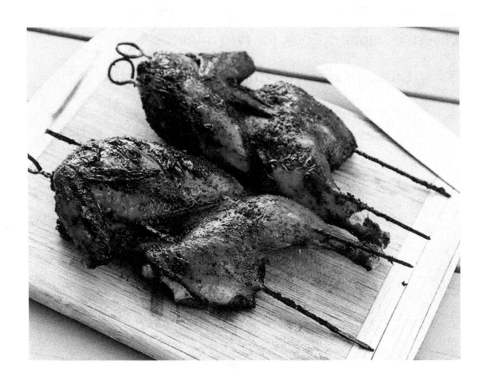

Total Prep & Cooking Time: Four hours and fifteen minutes

Yields: Six servings

Nutrition Facts: Calories: 311.2 | Protein: 30.7g | Carbs: 5.1g | Fat: 17.2g | Fiber: 0.8g

Ingredients

- One bunch of cilantro
- Three garlic cloves (peeled)
- Three red chili peppers (chopped)
- One tsp. of each
- Curry powder
- Turmeric (ground)
- One tbsp. of white sugar
- One pinch of salt
- Three tbsps. of fish sauce
- Three pounds of chicken (cut in small pieces)
- One-fourth cup of coconut milk

Method:

1.   Combine the cilantro, chili peppers, garlic, curry powder, turmeric, salt, and sugar in a food processor. Add the fish sauce and keep blending until smooth.

2.   Add the paste to the chicken and marinate for three hours.

3.   Heat a grill pan. Grease it with some oil.

4.   Add the chicken pieces to the grill. Brush them with coconut milk. Cook for fifteen minutes and turn in between. Cook until the chicken pieces are tender.

5.   Serve immediately.

Breaded Chicken Fillet

Total Prep & Cooking Time: One hour
Yields: Ten servings
Nutrition Facts: Calories: 201.3 | Protein: 30.6g | Carbs: 12.6g | Fat: 2.5g | Fiber: 2.6g

Ingredients

- Ten chicken breast halves

- Four green chili peppers (chopped)

- Five green onions (chopped)

- One tbsp. of lime zest

- Two limes (juiced)

- Three-fourth cup of cilantro

- Three tbsps. of fish sauce

- One lemongrass

- One tsp. of salt

- Two tsps. of white sugar

- One and a half tbsp. of each

- Parmesan cheese (grated)

- Dijon mustard

- Sesame seeds (toasted)

- One cup of bread crumbs

- Pepper and salt (for seasoning)

Method:

1. Combine green onions, peppers, lime juice, lime zest, half of the cilantro, lemongrass, fish sauce, sugar, salt, and mustard in a blender. Keep blending until smooth.

2. Cut the chicken into the desired size. Pour the marinade and combine it. Marinate for forty minutes.

3. Mix cilantro, breadcrumbs, cheese, salt, and sesame seeds in a bowl. Roll the chicken pieces in the mixture.

4. Add the chicken pieces in a greased baking tray. Bake them for twenty minutes at 175 degrees Celsius.

GkaiKamin

Total Prep & Cooking Time: Four hours and fifteen minutes
Yields: Four servings
Nutrition Facts: Calories: 402.3 | Protein: 37.9g | Carbs: 10.2g | Fat: 20.7g | Fiber: 2.8g

Ingredients

- One whole chicken

- Two stalks of lemongrass

- Twelve garlic cloves

- Two tbsps. of salt

- Five tbsps. of fresh turmeric (peeled, chopped)

- One tsp. of white peppercorns

Method:

1. Pound salt, lemongrass, turmeric, garlic, and pepper in a mortar and pestle. Make a very fine paste.

2. Cut the chicken lengthwise. Separate it into two pieces. Rub the chicken with the spice mix. Marinate for four hours in the refrigerator.

3. Grill the chicken for fifteen minutes.

4. Serve hot.

Thai-Style Sweet Chicken Bowl

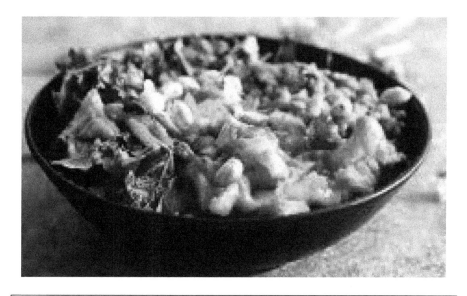

Total Prep & Cooking Time: Fifty-five minutes

Yields: Six servings

Nutrition Facts: Calories: 624.5 | Protein: 20.6g | Carbs: 89.6g | Fat: 23.6g | Fiber: 4.7g

Ingredients

- Three tbsps. of water

- One tsp. of salt

- Three chicken breast halves

- Half cup of soy sauce

- One can of coconut milk

- One cup of white sugar

- Two tbsps. of curry powder

- One mango (diced)

- Two and a half cup of clover sprouts

- One-third cup of cashews (chopped)

- One bunch of cilantro (chopped)

- Four green onions (chopped)

Method:

1.   Add the chicken breasts in a pan along with soy sauce and one tbsp. of water. Cover and cook for twenty minutes. Cut the cooked chicken into cubes.

2.   Mix sugar, coconut milk, and curry powder in a small saucepan. Simmer the mixture and add the mango cubes. Cook for five minutes.

3.   Serve the chicken in serving plates and top with cilantro, cashews, sprouts, and green onions. Drizzle the mango sauce from the top.

Chicken Panang Curry

Total Prep & Cooking Time: Thirty-five minutes

Yields: Four servings

Nutrition Facts: Calories: 590.1 | Protein: 19.6g | Carbs: 16.2g | Fat: 52.3g | Fiber: 3.6g

Ingredients

- One tbsp. of vegetable oil
- One-fourth cup of Panang curry paste
- Four cups of coconut milk
- Ten ounces of chicken breast (cubed)
- Two tbsps. of each
- Fish sauce
- Palm sugar
- Six leaves of kaffir lime (torn)
- Two red chili peppers (sliced)

- One bunch of basil leaves

Method:

1.   Take a large wok and heat the oil in it. Add the curry paste and cook for five minutes. Add the coconut milk along with the chicken. Cook for five minutes. Add the palm sugar, lime leaves, and fish sauce. Simmer for five minutes.

2.   Serve with basil and red chili peppers from the top.

Tamarind Chicken

> **Total Prep & Cooking Time: Twenty-five minutes**
>
> **Yields: Two servings**
>
> **Nutrition Facts: Calories: 445.2 | Protein: 42.3g | Carbs: 24.6g | Fat: 16.2g | Fiber: 1.3g**

Ingredients

- Three tbsps. of soy sauce

- Four tsps. of flour

- Fourteen ounces of chicken breast (cut in bite-size pieces)

For the tamarind sauce:

- One-third cup of water

- Two tbsps. of each

- Brown sugar

- Fish sauce

- Tamarind paste

- Olive oil

- Three garlic cloves (minced)

- One green chili pepper

- Half tsp. of ginger (grated)

Method:

1. Combine the flour and soy sauce in a bowl. Add the chicken and coat well.

2. Combine fish sauce, water, tamarind paste, and brown sugar in a bowl.

3. Heat the oil in a large wok. Add the chili pepper, garlic, and ginger. Cook for three minutes. Add the chicken and cook for two minutes.

4. Add half of the tamarind mixture and stir-fry for three minutes. Add the remaining sauce and cook for fifteen minutes.

5. Serve hot.

KhaiYat Sai (Thai Mushroom Stuffed Omelet)

> **Total Prep & Cooking Time: Thirty minutes**
>
> **Yields: Two servings**
>
> **Nutrition Facts: Calories: 223.6 | Protein: 16.5g | Carbs: 12.3g | Fat: 10.7g | Fiber: 3.2g**

Ingredients

- Half cup of mushrooms (sliced)

- Four scallions (chopped)

- One garlic clove (minced)

- Two sprigs of cilantro

- One Thai chili

- Two sprigs of Thai basil

- One tbsp. of tomato paste

- Four large eggs

- Two tbsps. of each
- Fish sauce
- Sesame seeds (black)
- Oyster sauce
- Vegetable oil
- Pepper and salt (for seasoning)

Method:

1.   Take a frying pan and heat the oil. Add the mushrooms and sauté for two minutes. Add the remaining veggies and cook for two minutes. Add pepper and salt for seasoning along with the tomato paste.

2.   Whisk the eggs along with sesame seeds, fish sauce, and chili.

3.   Add the egg mixture to the pan and cook for two minutes on each side. Fold the omelet in half. Cook for two minutes.

4.   Divide the omelet into two plates and serve hot with oyster sauce from the top.

KhaiLukKhoei (Son-In-Law Egg)

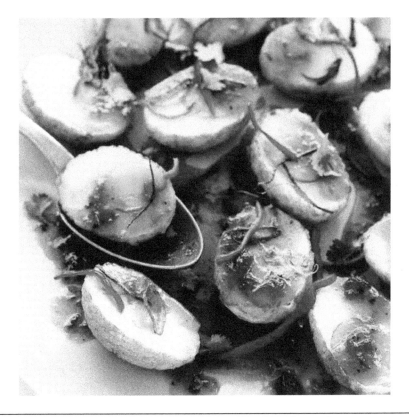

Total Prep & Cooking Time: One hour

Yields: Four servings

Nutrition Facts: Calories: 570.2 | Protein: 7.6g | Carbs: 24.6g | Fat: 47.6g | Fiber: 1.1g

Ingredients

- Eight boiled eggs (peeled)

- Half cup of shallots (fried)

- One cup of palm sugar (grated)

- One-fourth cup of fish sauce

- Two tbsps. of tamarind pulp

- Three tbsps. of water

- Two red chilies (sliced)

- Cilantro leaves (for garnishing)

- Vegetable oil (for frying)

Method:

1. Heat the oil in a large wok. Add the boiled eggs and fry them for five minutes. Remove the eggs and keep aside.

2. Take a pan and combine palm sugar, fish sauce, red chilies, tamarind pulp, and water. Simmer for three minutes.

3. Cut the fried eggs in half. Pour the prepared sauce over the halved eggs. Top with fried shallots.

4. Serve with cilantro from the top.

Hoi Tod (Egg Pancakes With Mussels)

Total Prep & Cooking Time: Thirty minutes

Yields: Two servings

Nutrition Facts: Calories: 73.2 | Protein: 7.6g | Carbs: 5.3g | Fat: 4.6g | Fiber: 0.3g

Ingredients

- One cup of mussels (cooked)

- Half cup of bean sprouts

- Two tsps. of soy sauce

- One tsp. of fish sauce

- Two spring onions (chopped)

- One large egg

- Three tbsps. of cooking oil

- Two coriander stalks

For the pancake mixture:

- One-third cup of corn flour

- One and a half cup of flour

- Two cups of rice flour

- Five cups of water

Method:

1.   Mix all the pancake mixture ingredients in a bowl. Make sure the consistency is loose and runny.

2.   Heat a pan and add twp tbsps. of oil. Add some of the pancake mixture and swirl the pan for covering.

3.   Arrange eight mussels on the pancake. Beat one egg along with some spring onions.

4.   Add the egg mixture over the mussels. Cook for two minutes on each side. Flip carefully.

5.   Sauté the bean sprouts in another pan for one minute. Add the fish sauce and soy sauce.

6.   Serve the bean sprouts on the plates and top with the pancakes.

KhaiYat Say (Thai Stuffed Egg)

Total Prep & Cooking Time: Thirty minutes

Yields: Two servings

Nutrition Facts: Calories: 430.3 | Protein: 12.6g | Carbs: 68.6g | Fat: 12.4g | Fiber: 3.9g

---

Ingredients

- Two large eggs

- Pepper and salt (for seasoning)

- Two tbsps. of each

- Carrot (diced)

- Green peas

- Onions (minced)

- One garlic clove (minced)

- One-hundred grams of pork (minced)

- One tbsp. of spring onions (minced)

- One tsp. of fish sauce

Method:

1. Heat oil in a wok. Add the carrots along with the onions.

2. Add the garlic. Cook for two minutes. Add the pork. Cook for five minutes.

3. Beat the eggs in a bowl. Add pepper and salt.

4. Remove the mince mixture from the wok and add the eggs.

5. Add the mince mixture to the center of the omelet. Fold the omelet from the sides.

6. Cook for two minutes.

Thai-Style Devilled Egg

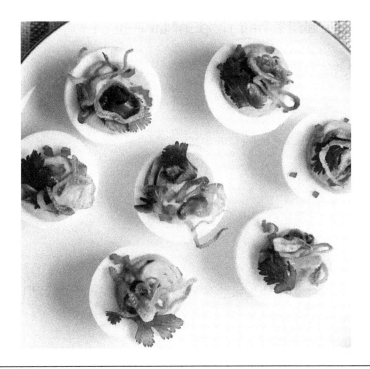

Total Prep & Cooking Time: Thirty minutes

Yields: Sixteen servings

Nutrition Facts: Calories: 73.2 | Protein: 7.7g |
Carbs: 5.1g | Fat: 6.8g | Fiber: 0.7g

Ingredients

- Eight large eggs (boiled, peeled)

- One tbsp. of sriracha sauce

- Two tbsps. of mayonnaise

- One and a half tbsp. of lime juice

- Two tsps. of fish sauce

- Red chili (sliced, for serving)

- Lime wedges (for serving)

Method:

1. Halve the eggs. Remove the egg yolks and keep in a bowl.

2. Add mayonnaise, sriracha sauce, fish sauce, and lime juice to the egg yolks. Use a spoon for mashing the yolks.

3. Spoon the mixture into the egg shells.

4. Serve with red chili and lime wedges from the top.

Pad Thai Egg Roll

Total Prep & Cooking Time: Forty-five minutes

Yields: Four servings

Nutrition Facts: Calories: 540.3 | Protein: 28.9g | Carbs: 27.3g | Fat: 27.6g | Fiber: 9.1g

Ingredients

- Hundred grams of rice noodles

- Two tbsps. of lemon juice

- One tbsp. of fish sauce

- Half tbsp. of brown sugar

- Two and a half tbsp. of kecapmanis

- Three tbsps. of peanut oil

- Three-hundred grams of tofu (firm, cut in one-inch pieces)

- One carrot (ribboned)

- Half cup of green beans (chopped)

- Three green onions (sliced)

- Eight large eggs

Method:

1.   Soak the noodles in hot water. Soak for ten minutes.

2.   Mix fish sauce, sugar, lemon juice, and half of the kecapmanis in a bowl.

3.   Take a wok and heat some oil in it. Add the tofu along with beans, carrots, and onions. Cook for two minutes. Add the mixture of lemon juice. Add the noodles and stir.

4.   Whisk the eggs in a bowl with two tbsps. of water.

5.   Add two tsps. of oil in the wok. Add one tbsp. of the egg mixture and swirl for making a round. Repeat with the remaining batter.

6.   Arrange the omelets on a plate. Add the noodle mixture in the center and roll the omelets.

7.   Serve with coriander from the top.

Chapter 3: Seafood Recipes

Shrimp Red Curry

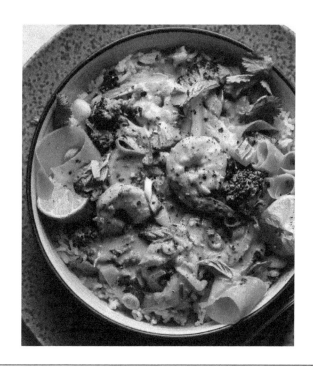

Total Prep & Cooking Time: Forty Minutes

Yields: Four servings

Nutrition Facts: Calories: 429.9 | Protein: 14.5g |
Carbs: 7.8g | Fat: 44.8g | Fiber: 2.8g

Ingredients

- Two cans of coconut milk

- Two tbsps. of red curry paste

- One tbsp. of fish sauce

- One hot chili pepper (minced)

- Twenty-four shrimps

Method:

1. Take a large wok and mix curry paste, coconut milk, minced pepper, and fish sauce. Simmer the mixture on low flame for ten minutes.

2. Add the shrimps and cook for fifteen minutes.

3. Serve hot with rice.

Thai Monkfish Curry

Total Prep & Cooking Time: One hour
Yields: Three servings
Nutrition Facts: Calories: 410.3 | Protein: 21.3g | Carbs: 10.6g | Fat: 35.1g | Fiber: 3.7g

Ingredients

- One tbsp. of peanut oil

- Half onion (chopped)

- One red bell pepper (chopped)

- Three tbsps. of curry paste

- One can of coconut milk

- Twelve ounces of monkfish

- One tbsp. of fish sauce

- Two tbsps. of each

- Lime juice

- Cilantro (chopped)

Method:

1.   Heat the peanut oil in a large pan. Add the onions and cook for five minutes.

2.   Add the red bell pepper. Cook for five minutes.

3.   Add the curry paste and mix well. Add the coconut milk and stir.

4.   Simmer the mixture for two minutes.

5.   Add the cubes of monkfish and simmer the curry for ten minutes. Add the lime juice and fish sauce. Cook for two minutes.

6.   Serve hot with rice.

Grilled Prawns and Spicy Lime-Peanut Vinaigrette

Total Prep & Cooking Time: One hour and twenty minutes

Yields: Eight servings

Nutrition Facts: Calories: 530.9 | Protein: 28.9g | Carbs: 14.6g | Fat: 30.7g | Fiber: 2.2g

Ingredients

- One-fourth cup of each
- Lemongrass
- Galangal root (minced)
- Lime juice
- Mirin sauce
- Vinegar
- Two tbsps. of garlic (minced)

- One-fourth tbsp. of cilantro

- One green chili (minced)

- Three-fourth cup of peanut oil

- Two pounds of shrimp

- Three tbsps. of lime zest

- Two tsps. of fish sauce

- Two Thai green chilies (minced)

- Two and a half tsp. of garlic (minced)

- Half cup of peanut butter

- One-third cup of peanut oil

- One tbsp. of cilantro (chopped)

- Three-fourth cup of peanuts (roasted)

- One pinch of salt

Method:

1. Combine half of the ginger, lemongrass, cilantro, garlic, oil, and one minced chili. Add the shrimps and toss for coating. Marinate the shrimps for thirty minutes.

2.   Heat a grill pan.

3.   Add lime juice, mirin, vinegar, soy sauce, and water in a food processor. Add one tbsp. of ginger, two chili peppers, fish sauce, lime zest, peanut butter, and garlic. Blend the ingredients until smooth. Slowly add peanut oil while blending. Add cilantro and chopped peanuts. Keep aside.

4.   Grill the marinated shrimps for two minutes on each side.

5.   Serve the grilled shrimps with vinaigrette by the side.

Steamed Crab Leg With Lemongrass

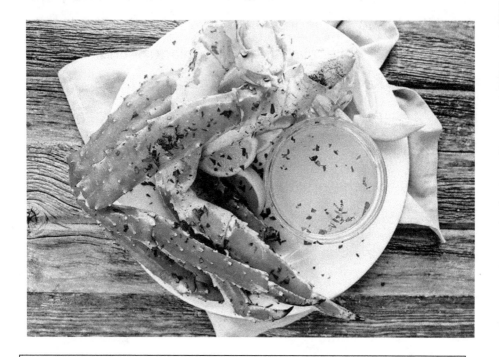

Total Prep & Cooking Time: Thirty minutes

Yields: Two servings

Nutrition Facts: Calories: 580.6 | Protein: 87.3g | Carbs: 5.1g | Fat: 19.2g | Fiber: 0.6g

Ingredients

- Two tbsps. of oil

- Three garlic cloves (minced)

- One-inch of galangal

- One stalk of lemongrass

- Two and a half tbsp. of fish sauce

- One tbsp. of oyster sauce

- One pinch of salt

- Two pounds of crab legs (cooked)

Method:

1.   Take a large pot and heat it over medium heat. Add the oil.

2.   Add ginger, garlic, and lemongrass to the oil. Cook for two minutes. Add the oyster sauce, fish sauce, pepper, and salt.

3.   Add the legs of crab and cook for fifteen minutes. Stir well.

4.   Serve hot.

Grilled Mahi Mahi With Thai Coconut Sauce

> **Total Prep & Cooking Time: Thirty minutes**
>
> **Yields: Two servings**
>
> **Nutrition Facts: Calories: 490.2 | Protein: 31.6g | Carbs: 8.6g | Fat: 32.6g | Fiber: 2.8g**

Ingredients

- Two cups of coconut milk

- Two tbsps. of cilantro (chopped)

- Three tbsps. of scallions (chopped)

- Two and a half tbsp. of lime juice

- Four tsps. of ginger (grated)

- Two garlic cloves (minced)

- One tsp. of fish sauce

- Two fillets of mahi-mahi

Method:

1.   Heat the grill pan.

2.   Add cilantro, coconut milk, scallions, garlic, lime juice, ginger, and fish sauce in a medium-sized saucepan. Boil the mixture.

3.   Brush the fillets of mahi-mahi with the prepared sauce. Boil the remaining sauce until thickened.

4.   Add the fillets of mahi-mahi to the grill pan. Cook for seven minutes on each side.

5.   Serve the grilled fish fillets with sauce from the top.

Thai-Style Green Curry Prawns

Total Prep & Cooking Time: Forty minutes

Yields: Four servings

Nutrition Facts: Calories: 530.2 | Protein: 21.7g | Carbs: 16.6g | Fat: 40.3g | Fiber: 7.9g

Ingredients

- Half tsp. of cumin
- One and a half tsp. of coriander seeds
- One tbsp. of ginger (grated)
- Four tsps. of garlic (minced)
- Two green chili peppers
- Three stalks of lemongrass
- One-third cup of cilantro
- Two tbsps. of lime juice

- One tbsp. of lime zest

- Three tbsps. of oil

- Half pound of beans

- One can of baby corn

- One-fourth tbsp. of soy sauce

- One can of coconut milk

- Three-fourth pounds of shrimp

Method:

1. Add ginger, coriander, cumin, green chili peppers, garlic, cilantro, lemongrass, lime zest, lime juice, and two tbsps. of oil in a high power blender. Blend for making a smooth paste.

2. Add the remaining oil in an iron skillet. Add the beans along with the baby corns. Cook for thirty seconds.

3. Add the prepared paste, coconut milk, and soy sauce. Boil the mixture.

4. Simmer for seven minutes and add the shrimps.

5. Cook for five minutes.

6. Serve hot with rice.

Thai Fried Prawns With White Pepper and Garlic

Ingredients

- Eight garlic cloves (minced)
- Two tbsps. of flour
- Three tbsps. of fish sauce
- Two and a half tbsp. of soy sauce
- One tbsp. of sugar
- Half tsp. of white pepper
- One-fourth cup of oil
- One pound of shrimp

Method:

1.   Mix garlic, flour, soy sauce, fish sauce, white pepper, and sugar in a large bowl. Add the prawns for coating.

2.   Heat the oil in a pan. Add the prawns. Cook for two minutes.

3.   Serve hot.

Thai Clam and Shrimp Curry

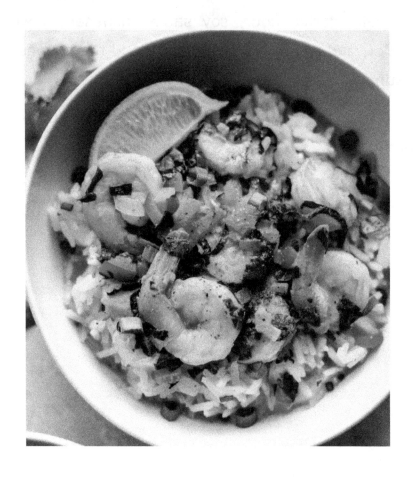

Total Prep & Cooking Time: Forty-five minutes

Yields: Four servings

Nutrition Facts: Calories: 320.6 | Protein: 11.6g |
Carbs: 12.5g | Fat: 27.3g | Fiber: 3.2g

Ingredients

- Two tbsps. of oil

- One onion (chopped)

- One red bell pepper

- One tbsp. of ginger (minced)

- Two garlic cloves (minced)

- One tsp. of chili paste

- One can of coconut milk

- Four large clams

- One-fourth cup of chicken stock

- One tsp. of each

- Brown sugar

- Fish sauce

- Three tbsps. of basil

- Twelve shrimps

- One lime

Method:

1. Heat oil in a large pan. Add red bell pepper and onion. Cook for four minutes. Add garlic and ginger. Cook for two minutes.

2. Add the chili paste along with coconut milk. Stir well.

3. Add the clams. Cook for five minutes. Grate some zest from the lime and mix. Add some lemon juice.

4. Add the shrimp and basil. Cook for ten minutes. Add chicken stock for adjusting the consistency.

5. Remove the clams.

6. Serve the curry with basil and lime zest.

Whole Fried Tilapia With Chilies and Basil

Total Prep & Cooking Time: Thirty-five minutes

Yields: Four servings

Nutrition Facts: Calories: 330.3 | Protein: 14.6g | Carbs: 9.6g | Fat: 31.3g | Fiber: 1.6g

Ingredients

- One whole tilapia fish
- Oil for frying
- Five red chili peppers
- Six garlic cloves (minced)
- One onion (chopped)
- Two tbsps. of each
- Soy sauce
- Fish sauce

- One-fourth cup of each

- Cilantro (chopped)

- Basil (chopped)

Method:

1. Heat the oil in a large pan.

2. Clean the fish and make various slits on it using a sharp knife.

3. Add the fish to the oil. Fry for ten minutes. Remove from the oil. Drain excess oil.

4. Heat some oil in a skillet and add garlic, onion, and chili peppers. Cook for seven minutes.

5. Add soy sauce and fish sauce. Add cilantro and basil. Mix well.

6. Serve the fish on a plate and pour the prepared sauce all over the fish.

Chapter 4: Snacks & Dessert Recipes

Thai Crab Cake

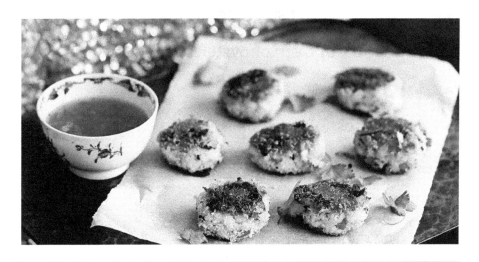

Total Prep & Cooking Time: Thirty minutes

Yields: Four servings

**Nutrition Facts: Calories: 68.6 | Protein: 5.6g |
Carbs: 6.2g | Fat: 2.2g | Fiber: 0.5g**

Ingredients

- Eight ounces of crab meat

- Three spring onions (sliced)

- Three lime leaves (thinly sliced)

- One chili (minced)

- One tbsp. of lime juice

- Two tbsps. of fish sauce

- One-fourth tbsp. of oyster sauce

- Three large eggs

- Two tsps. of mayonnaise

- Two cups of panko bread crumbs

- Half tsp. of garlic salt

- One cup of oil

Method:

1.   Add crab meat, lime leaves, onions, chili, fish sauce, lime juice, one egg, oyster sauce, half cup of panko bread crumbs, and mayonnaise in a blender.

Process the ingredients for two minutes. You can add more bread crumbs if needed.

2.   Make cakes from the mixture using your hands. Keep aside.

3.   Break the remaining eggs in a bowl. Whisk the eggs.

4.   Add bread crumbs and garlic salt in a dish. Mix well.

5.   Dip the prepared crab cakes in the whisked eggs and then coat them in the bread crumbs mixture.

6.   Heat oil in a pan. Add the crab cakes. Fry for two minutes on each side.

7.   Serve hot.

Thai Sticky Meatballs

Total Prep & Cooking Time: Thirty-five minutes

Yields: Six servings

Nutrition Facts: Calories: 330.2 | Protein: 17.6g | Carbs: 21.3g | Fat: 16.5g | Fiber: 0.9g

Ingredients

For the meatballs:

- One cup of bread crumbs

- One large egg

- One tbsp. of green curry paste

- One tsp. of each

- Ginger paste

- Garlic paste

- One-fourth tsp. of salt

- One and a half tbsp. of fish sauce

- Five-hundred grams of beef (ground)

For the sauce:

- Two tbsps. of each

- Sweet chili sauce

- Soy sauce

- Honey

- One tbsp. of rice vinegar

- Two chilies (chopped)

- Half cup of water

- One tsp. of corn flour

Method:

1. Preheat your oven at two-hundred degrees Celsius.

2. Mix all the listed ingredients for the meatballs except for the beef. Add the ground beef and mix well.

3.   Make twenty balls from the beef mixture. Place them on a baking sheet. Bake for twenty-five minutes.

4.   Whisk the sauce ingredients in a bowl. Add the sauce to a wok and warm for two minutes.

5.   Add the meatballs and toss them in the sauce.

6.   Serve hot.

Red Curry Puffs

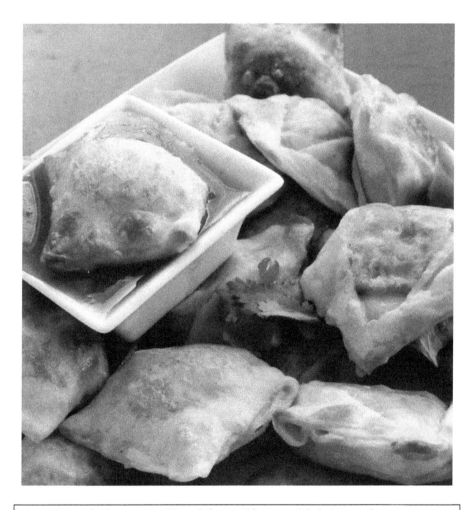

Total Prep & Cooking Time: Thirty minutes

Yields: Four servings

Nutrition Facts: Calories: 180.6 | Protein: 5.6g | Carbs: 24.8g | Fat: 6.6g | Fiber: 0.4g

Ingredients

For the filling:

- One medium-sized potato
- One tbsp. of each
- Fish sauce
- Soy sauce
- One tsp. of each
- Red curry paste
- Chili paste
- Four tbsps. of each
- Corn
- Peas

For the wrappers:

- One egg white
- Thirty wonton wrappers
- One tbsp. of each
- Olive oil
- Cornstarch

- Two tbsps. of water

Method:

1. Start by boiling the potato.

2. Combine cornstarch and water in a bowl.

3. Mash the potato and mix it with curry paste, peas, soy sauce, chili paste, and fish sauce. Make a fine paste.

4. Heat your oven and two-hundred degrees Celsius.

5. Take the wonton wrappers and line the borders with the cornstarch mixture.

6. Add one tsp. of the paste in the middle of each wrapper and fold them in a triangle shape.

7. Combine egg white with one tsp. of water. Brush the filled wrappers with the mixture.

8. Bake the puffs in the oven for ten minutes.

9. Serve hot.

Thai Mango Pudding

Total Prep & Cooking Time: Two hours and thirty minutes
Yields: Four servings
Nutrition Facts: Calories: 251.3 | Protein: 4.2g | Carbs: 31.3g | Fat: 14.6g | Fiber: 3.2g

Ingredients

- Two ripe mangoes

- One packet of gelatin

- Half a cup of hot water

- One-third cup of white sugar

- One cup of coconut milk

Method:

1.   Scoop out the mango flesh and add it to a blender. Puree the mango flesh.

2.   Heat some oil in pan two minutes. Remove the pan from heat. Add the gelatin. Mix well.

3.   Add white sugar to the mixture of gelatin.

4.   Add the gelatin mixture to the prepared mango puree. Add the coconut milk and combine.

5.   Pour the prepared mango mixture into bowls. Refrigerate for two hours.

Thai Crème Caramel

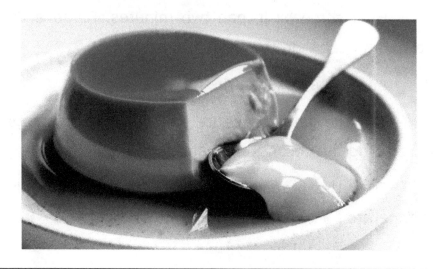

Total Prep & Cooking Time: Thirty-five minutes

Yields: Four servings

Nutrition Facts: Calories: 205.6 | Protein: 5.1g | Carbs: 26.2g | Fat: 10.3g | Fiber: 0.2g

Ingredients

- One cup of coconut milk

- Two large eggs

- One tbsp. of sugar

- One-fourth tsp. of pandan paste

- One-fourth cup of Thai palm sugar

- One pinch of salt

- One tsp. of coconut oil

Method:

1. Preheat your oven at one-hundred and seventy-five degrees Celsius.

2. Grease four ramekins using oil.

3. Beat the eggs using a fork. Add sugar, salt, pandan paste, and coconut milk. Mix well.

4. Add palm sugar at the bottom of each ramekin.

5. Pour the prepared mixture into the ramekins.

6. Arrange the ramekins on a baking dish. Add some water for covering one-fourth of the ramekins.

7. Bake for thirty minutes.

8. Chill the ramekins for five minutes.

9. Use a sharp knife for running along the inside wall of ramekins.

10. Overturn the loosened ramekins on serving plates.

11. Serve immediately.

Thai-Style Iced Coffee

Total Prep & Cooking Time: One hour and ten minutes

Yields: Four servings

Nutrition Facts: Calories: 110.3 | Protein: 3.2g | Carbs: 16.9g | Fat: 4.1g | Fiber: 0.2g

Ingredients

- Two large cups of brewed coffee

- Six tbsps. of condensed milk

- One-third cup of ice cubes

- One-fourth cup of heavy cream

Method:

1.   Pour the coffee in a jug. Add condensed milk. Stir well for mixing. Add a few cubes of ice and refrigerate for one hour.

2.   Pour the iced coffee in glasses with ice cubes. Add heavy cream from the top.

Thai Tapioca Pudding

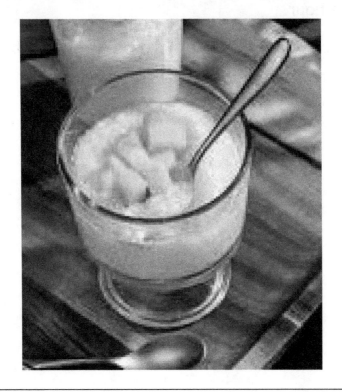

Total Prep & Cooking Time: Thirty minutes

Yields: Four servings

Nutrition Facts: Calories: 310.3 | Protein: 2.1g |
Carbs: 1.3g | Fat: 5.6g | Fiber: 0.3g

Ingredients

- Half cup of tapioca

- Three cups of water

- One-eighth tsp. of salt

- One can of coconut milk

- One mango (sliced)

- Maple syrup (for serving)

Method:

1. Cover tapioca with one and a half cups of water in a bowl. Soak for twenty minutes.

2. Combine salt, tapioca, and two cups of water in a bowl. Boil the mixture and simmer for ten minutes.

3. Let the mixture sit for ten minutes.

4. Refrigerate the mixture for thirty minutes.

5. For serving, scoop out one-fourth cup of tapioca in serving bowls. Add one-third cup of coconut milk. Stir for mixing.

6. Garnish with mango slices and maple syrup.

Mangosteen Clafouti

Total Prep & Cooking Time: One hour and ten minutes

Yields: Six servings

Nutrition Facts: Calories: 165.3 | Protein: 5.6g | Carbs: 23.1g | Fat: 5.6g | Fiber: 0.6g

Ingredients

- Five mangosteen fruit
- Two tbsps. of sugar
- One tsp. of cornstarch
- One-third cup of rice flour
- Four eggs
- One pinch of salt
- One cup of coconut milk
- One-third tsp. of each
- Vanilla extract
- Lemon peel (grated)

- Coconut extract

Method:

1.   Preheat your oven at one-hundred and seventy-five degrees Celsius.

2.   Grease six ramekins with oil.

3.   Use a knife for removing the stem section of the fruits. Remove the skin. Remove the white segments of the fruit.

4.   Toss the fruit with one tbsp. of sugar and cornstarch.

5.   Arrange the fruit segments at the bottom of the ramekins.

6.   Whisk eggs with sugar and salt in a bowl. Add flour and mix well.

7.   Add lemon peel, coconut milk, coconut extract, and vanilla extract. Mix well.

8.   Pour the mixture into each ramekin.

9.   Place the ramekins in a baking dish. Pour two cups of water in the dish.

10.   Bake for one hour.

Dragon Fruit Martini

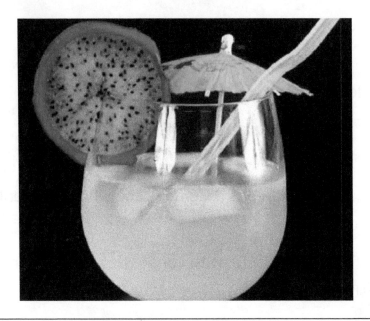

Total Prep & Cooking Time: Twelve minutes
Yields: Two servings
Nutrition Facts: Calories: 121.3 | Protein: 1.1g | Carbs: 10.2g | Fat: 3.2g | Fiber: 0.9g

Ingredients

- One dragon fruit (ripe)
- Half cup of vodka

- One tbsp. of lime juice

- Three tbsps. of white sugar

- Four ice cubes

- One-fourth cup of coconut milk

Method:

1.   Scoop out the flesh of the dragon fruit.

2.   Add the fruit flesh in a blender. Add the remaining ingredients. Blend for one minute.

3.   Serve the chilled martini in glasses and garnish with small pieces of dragon fruit.

Conclusion

I hope you enjoyed this journey into international Thai cuisine, and got a taste of the true flavor of oriental dishes, with the ingredients and preparation of the best Thai Chefs.

Have you tried these dishes to impress your guests?

and your family?

Pack your bags for your next trip, I will make you taste new fantastic recipes!!!

Thanks for coming with me and see you soon.

CPSIA information can be obtained
at www.ICGtesting.com
Printed in the USA
BVHW012219230321
603253BV00004B/95